THE DOLCE DIET

COLLEGE DIET GUIDE

By MIKE DOLCE
with Brandy Roon

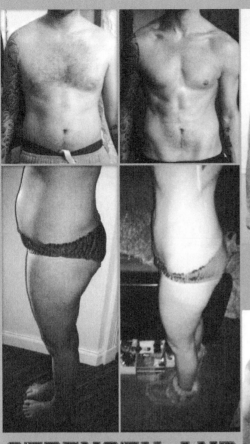

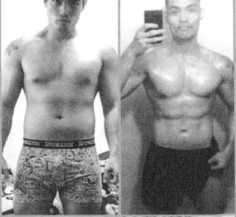

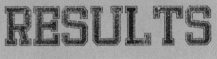

STRENGTH AND
PASSION

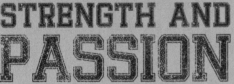

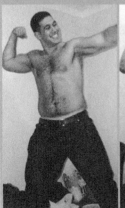

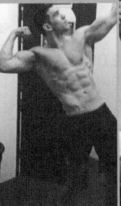

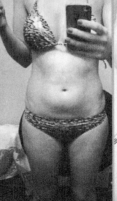

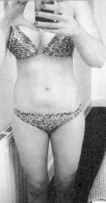

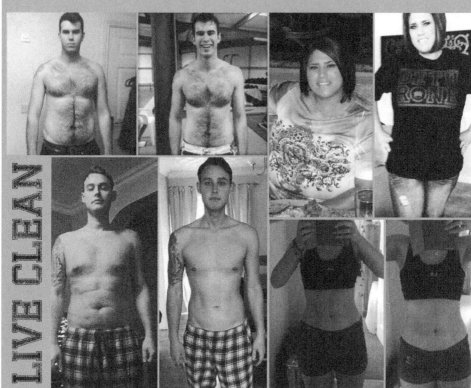

LIVE CLEAN

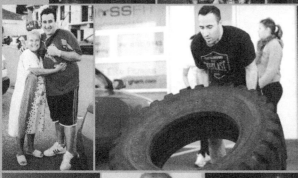

HAVE
SOME
FUN!

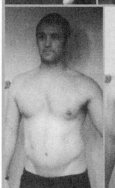
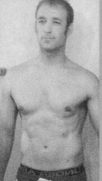
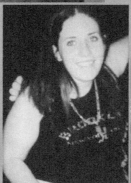
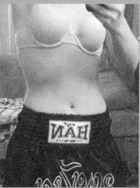

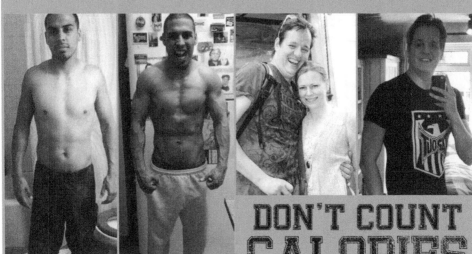

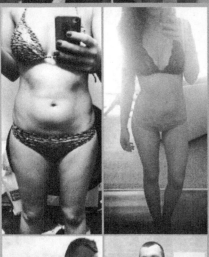

DON'T COUNT CALORIES

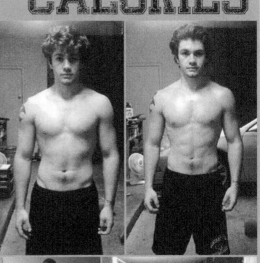

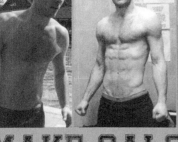

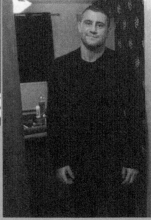

MAKE CALORIES COUNT!

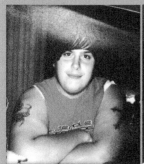
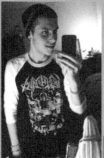

ORGANIC

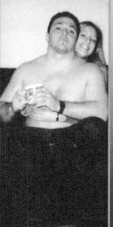
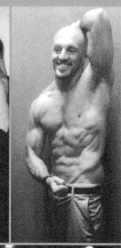

EARTH-GROWN
NUTRIENTS

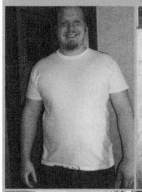
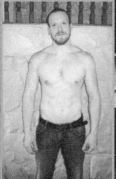

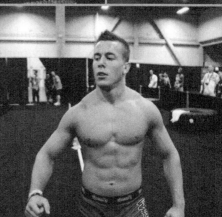

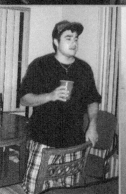
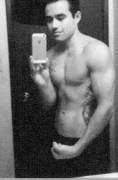

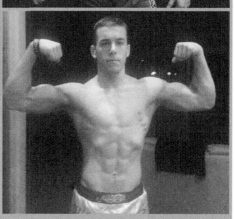

WORK
HARD!

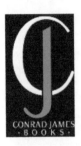

Conrad James Books
Las Vegas, NV
www.conradjamesbooks.com

Printed in the United States of America.
ISBN 978-0-9849631-7-1

Edited by Brandy Roon & Sarah Veit
Illustrations & Design by Brady Scott: **www.bradyscott.weebly.com**

Special thanks to:

Sean Kochel and Aaron Fried
for your tireless work in helping to put this book together.
All your nights of debauchery were not in vain.

Table of Contents

Epigraph
Introduction

THE DOLCE DIET

COLLEGE DIET GUIDE

By MIKE DOLCE
with Brandy Roon

EPIGRAPH

"A lion does not concern himself with the opinions of the sheep."
~*Tywin Lannister*, ***Game of Thrones***

Introduction

I coach the greatest athletes in the world – the elite of the elite. But they are no different than you or I. They simply make better choices. While you're sitting on your ass on a Saturday night eating pizza, drinking beer and illegally streaming the fights live on Pay-Per-View, they are...well, they are not. My athletes have goals that they stick to through discipline and hard work. They commit to tasks and hold themselves accountable. Life is full of choices but probably none so important as how you treat your body.

I don't know why it always surprises me when I see people lined up like cows to the slaughter at popular fast food chains. It plays out like a horror movie to me. No! Don't open the door! Don't order the number three! Don't get meat on top of meat on top of meat!
How do these folks arrive at the choice that that's the best thing to put into their bodies? How can they eat something and have no idea where it comes from or what anomalous parts make up the mystery meat? Because if they did, I can almost guarantee they wouldn't be eating it.

Luckily, college is about doing your own thing. It's about learning to live and think independently. Some colleges require incoming freshmen to have a meal plan, which might make you feel limited in your choices.

In fact, that's how we got the idea to write this guide. My cousin Sean was forced to buy a meal plan at his college and the healthy options, he says, were severely limited. He gained weight and felt terrible. He didn't know he could stock his room with healthy options and supplement, if not completely replace, the dining hall food with his own. We came up with a plan that included an exercise routine and easy, affordable recipes that helped him lose 55 lbs. in eight months.

When his friend Aaron saw Sean's transformation, he, too, jumped on board, learning all he could about how to best create a healthier lifestyle while living at school. Now you can do the same!

We've included recipes, exercises and lifestyle habits to help you be in the best shape possible while living at school, no matter the restrictions.
From the first meal, you will feel the difference! And you'll save money, and gain energy and strength (not to mention confidence)! And what's sexier than that!?

Living a Dolce Lifestyle is so easy and takes such little effort that anyone can do it! After all, our book series didn't become an international bestseller because it made a great coaster.

Template programs don't work. We're all so different, how could they? But the Dolce Diet Principles are so easy to tailor to your unique wants and needs that even a <ahem> college student can do it!

People all around the world have proven that these simple methods work! And now it's your turn to take control of your life! Before you even finish this book – in fact, in this very moment – your life will already be changed forever!

Keep your choices where they belong – in your own hands! You are an independent thinker. Even if you've never before cooked a thing, you can make the recipes in this book. And you can do it in your dorm with no kitchen at all. EASY!

This guide is about staying as healthy as possible while faced with the college grind. Your brain and body need clean fuel. You're there to be smart, make intelligent choices and take over the world.

And I'm here to help.

THE PROBLEM

"The good thing about the American dream is that you can
just go to sleep and try it all again the next day."
~*Michael Scott, The Office*

SEAN

Age: 22 • **Starting Weight:** 205 • **Current Weight:** 147

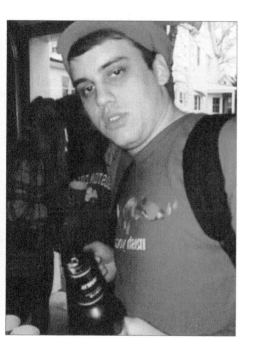 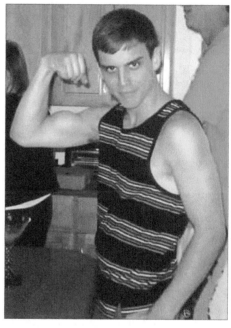

I hate cafeteria food. Some people love it. I look at it like the plague broke out all over the buffet's congealed Alfredo sauce – and not because I thought it was unhealthy – just because I didn't like it.

I also had no idea how to prepare healthy food (or any food for that matter) in my dorm. As you might imagine, my eating habits made my transition to college life somewhat difficult. To top it off, I was homesick. These issues manifested some pretty terrible eating habits.

I never skipped breakfast because I've always loved breakfast foods like eggs, pancakes, waffles and bagels, but lunch and dinner were often missed. I normally filled in these missing meals with either a granola bar or some variety of spreadable cheese and cracker snacks, and possibly a frozen peanut-butter and jelly sandwich if I was feeling especially daring. The times that I did manage to make it to the dining hall resulted in some pretty poor choices: pizza, French fries, a few cookies, a turkey sandwich, probably some pasta, and a few glasses of Gatorade was the usual meal for both lunch and dinner. Fortunately, I was so picky that I stayed away from some REALLY terrible foods that everyone seemed to enjoy (Ramen noodles, Mac N' Cheese, Mac N' Cheese mixed with gas station quality beef jerky, processed soups, etc.).

On top of bad dietary choices, I also fell victim to awful overall lifestyle choices. I drank beer heavily 3-4 times per week, and any class that began before 10am was routinely missed. I was still performing well in my classes, but there was always a stressful struggle between motivating myself to sit down and do my calculus home-work vs. drinking with some friends or going out to a party. Ultimately, I had to choose between the two opposing forces, but that comes a little later.

December of my freshman year sucked. My weight had increased from a decent 175 lbs. in my senior year of high school to a disgusting 205. My mood was just blah, my body was bloated, and I couldn't give a shit about most things.

This holiday break was like all the others, except for the minor detail that I was now A FATASS. That's right – my neck was huge, I was sprouting breasts, my stomach fell over my pants, and I had stretch marks down the sides of my hips. Needless to say, I was convinced during a trip to visit Mike and Brandy that I needed to start showing some real concern about where my life was headed and what the consequences of my actions would be.

I was on my way to becoming a character in WALL-E. I knew I had to make a change, or I needed to pick out the color of my future mode of transportation – a motorized scooter.

Mike gave me a copy of Living Lean to read on my flight home and said, "We love you, but if you come back here looking like you do now I'm going to leave you at bag-gage claim with all the other overstuffed luggage."
By the time my flight landed, I was a new man. Invigorated and empowered at how simple it was to make a change. The principles Mike teaches are so easy. You can't be any lazier than I was at this moment, and Mike made it so clear to me what I was do-ing to myself.
I'd been gorging on foods full of toxins, and I knew they had to go. How could I expect to perform to the best of my ability when I was slowly killing myself with pro-cessed foods?

I was surprised by how much weight I could lose by simply increasing my water intake. This really worked to boost my confidence, and it lit the path to my success. From here, I slowly began to implement more and more of the Dolce Diet Principles and made improvements in daily increments such as:

• **No more bacon in the omelet today**
• **Start bringing a snack to class every day**
• **Start working out again**

- Wake up early so that you aren't miserable in class at 8am
- Focus on eating earth-grown nutrients
- Drink less beer
- Sleep more

Six months later, in May of 2011, I was a slimmer 170 lbs., but I still wasn't happy. I had corrected a lot of my mistakes: no more drinking every night of the week, I ate three well-balanced meals a day and I exercised regularly. I flew out once again to see Mike and Brandy in Las Vegas, but this time, I had something to be proud of: I had lost 35 lbs. and still had room to lose more – and that is precisely what happened.

With a solid base and a newly written track record for success, I was able to apply more and more principles of healthy living to my everyday life.
I left Las Vegas weighing 150 lbs., which meant I had lost a total of 55 lbs. in about 8 months!

Today, as I begin my senior year, I stand at a lean 147 lbs. at 8 percent body fat. Everything is better about my life since I decided to become healthy and fit: My grades are spectacular, I can take on more tasks within a given space of time, I can do everything more efficiently, and of course what we are ultimately striving for – I am happy about life.

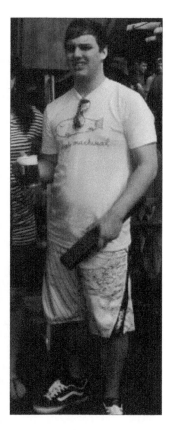
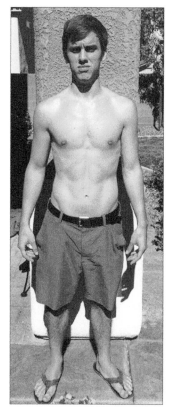

AARON

I've always been skinny. Even in my best periods of physical activity, I've never put on much muscle, and in my worst periods of bad diet and sitting around, I've never put on too much fat. But college living threw my mind and body into a spiral the likes of which I'd never known. It happened because I simply didn't know how to create a healthy routine.

In high school, my saving grace was my fast metabolism, and the fact that I still spent some time eating well and exercising a little. But all of that went out the window when I got to college, where I mismanaged my time while mistreating my body.

During freshman year, I ruined my sleep cycle, and basically became nocturnal. Most days, I'd wake up minutes before class – or sometimes sleep through class – then rush off on an empty stomach, not having a meal until mid-afternoon. I was starving by the time I ate, so I'd try to get the most food possible with one "lunch swipe" on my meal card – fried chicken tenders and French fries were a regular choice. Then I wouldn't get hungry again until late at night, when the dining halls were closed, and be forced to eat expensive-but-crappy food out of the microwave.

That's a routine of two horrible meals per day, with my "dinner" usually taking place an hour or two before midnight. On good days, I would force myself to have a proper routine and eat three meals a day and maybe exercise or play some intramural sports, but I didn't have the capability to make this my typical schedule. I had no energy because of the garbage I was eating.

When we go to the dining hall, most college students will grab whatever is fast, cheap and tasty. I resorted to toaster pizza saddled with processed cheese and dough that tasted like cardboard. I ate quesadillas filled with bright-orange "cheddar cheese" and rubbery chicken. Chicken patties were a favorite at my school's all-you-can-eat dining hall – which, after a little research, I found out were made by taking all of the parts of the chicken that can't be used for meat, throwing them in a blender with a bunch of artificial flavors, chemicals and some spices, then forming the resulting slimy goo into a patty-shape and breading it. To top it all off, it was cooked in the deep-fryer.

Gross. Imagine filling your body with that for an entire year? I did it for two years straight. (Spoiler: It doesn't end well.)

By sophomore year, my habits went from bad to worse. I was taking more difficult classes, which I couldn't afford to skip. So I forced myself to attend (almost) all of my classes, but didn't change any of my eating, sleeping or exercise habits. So I was sleepier in class, lazier outside of it, and ate even more erratically.

Typically, I would wake up just in time to rush to class, and afterward I'd return to my dorm, exhausted, to nap until my next class. When I stopped to grab breakfast, I'd pick up some bagels smeared with artificially flavored cream cheese. Without exercising, I was beginning to feel a strain on my body. I was only 20 years old and already feeling like I was 70. And when you feel lethargic, you only get lazier, which makes you more lethargic…and so on. In college, it's easy to get sucked into downward spirals like this.

I didn't feel energetic like I did in high school, and sometimes even going to class was draining. I knew that I had to be more active, so occasionally I'd drag myself out for a short run, or a trip to the gym, but I could still never turn it into a habit – how could I, while I kept abusing my body? I was being stupid about the way I slept, and more importantly, the way that I was eating.

I wasn't overweight, but I was starting to put on fat. I wasn't sick, but I sure as hell didn't feel healthy. My normal body weight at the beginning of college varied between 125 and 130 lbs. (see, I told you I'm a small guy), with my body fat usually around 12 percent. By the end of the year, for the first time in my life, I started to have visible areas of fat. I was growing a little gut, and there were even miniature "moobs" on my chest. I had a bit of a double-chin coming in. My weight was climbing toward 140 and my body fat was fast approaching 20 percent.

I knew something had to change. The summer after sophomore year, my friend Sean returned home with great results after spending a month visiting with Mike Dolce and his wife, Brandy, and I saw what I needed to do.

So a month before entering junior year, I read The Dolce Diet: Living Lean and immediately adopted its principles. I took a lot of important lessons from the book, and started turning the ship around, no longer lost at sea.

- **I cut out all processed foods.**
- **Snacks changed from chips and chocolate to almonds and berries.**
- **Every meal included some green vegetables.**
- **I realized that people can eat seeds, that they taste good, are packed with energy-inducing nutrients, and are some of the healthiest things to eat on the planet.**
- **Most importantly, I found a bunch of recipes that were both delicious and nutritious, and used that as my daily diet.**

The short-term results were quick and obvious. Some of the excess fat I'd put on over the past two years began melting away within a few weeks. My energy levels soared, and I felt capable of doing anything that I wanted to do. As a result, my attitude improved: I had gotten a taste of success, and I wanted a whole lot more.

By the beginning of my junior year, I was committed to keeping myself in good health. My room was stocked with some of the essentials: fruit and veggies were in my fridge, chia seeds and flaxseed were on my shelves, I had coconut oil to put in my coffee, and psyllium husk powder, just in case the dining hall served up something particularly nasty. I was exercising regularly, getting rid of the last bits of fat, and replacing it with muscle. I'm much more healthy and physically fit than I ever was.

I'm proof that The Dolce Diet isn't just for overweight people burning off lots of fat, or for highly muscular athletes – it's for anyone who wants a healthy lifestyle.

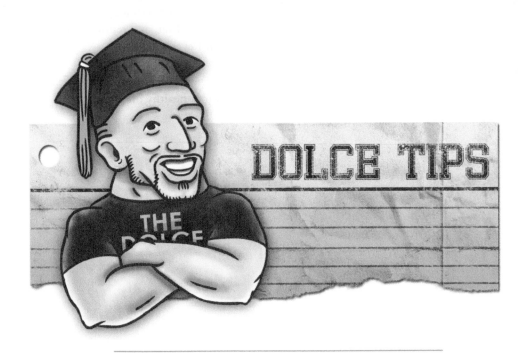

Tip: It takes the average person 14 minutes to fall asleep. Choose the time you need to wake up and plan to get 6-9 hours of sleep per night.

LEARNING THE HARD WAY

Sean and Aaron are just like you. The same challenges you face, they had to deal with. The first challenge is leaving home, which is awesome, but also requires you to start buying your own toilet paper. And for some, that means wiping your own ass for the first time.

The next challenge is overcoming the toxic food system in most colleges.
Did you know that nearly all college freshmen are required to purchase meal plans?

In Sean's case, that was $3,000 per semester, $6,000 per year. Even though Sean had a grocery store 5 minutes from campus, his parents already paid $6,000 to the college to feed him, and they weren't about to give him one cent more. To make matters worse, the menus most colleges provide are filled with highly processed, preserved and chemically contaminated food-type substances dressed up as pasta, burgers, fries and dressings.
Once Sean started following the Dolce Diet Principles and living lean, we calculated that his DOLCE meal plan cost him $800 per semester to completely feed himself earth-grown nutrients that he made with his own hands, and he was never hungry or felt sick. Talk about inexpensive! Now Sean was getting much greater nutrients at a dramatically lower cost, allowing him to buy the best possible options.

And you can do the same once you apply the simple lessons taught in this book! Not only will you establish the habits of eating well, I'll show you how to create the perfect environment for your success.
Eating healthy at college means anticipating every obstacle campus life will throw at you and busting right through it.

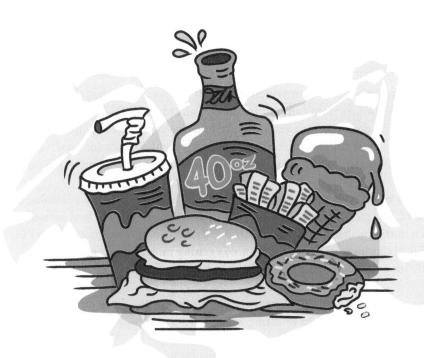

THE CAMPUS BLACKLIST

Don't Do These Things Unless You Want to #FAIL

Your college years are a time to explore your independence, test boundaries and push your limits! It's also the time you learn to take care of yourself! Here are some things to watch out for while you're having all the fun!

Focus on your goals, but don't forget to let loose every once in a while!

Vampirism – (Get Your Sleep!)

Sleep is the way your body recovers from the day-to-day wear and tear. If you want your brain to be so powerful it can shape steel into balloon animals with a single thought, it needs sleep! Many studies show that sleep deprivation has a negative effect on your mind. Lack of sleep can also break down your body, making it susceptible to storing body fat and breaking down muscle tissue. I like to set a sleep schedule using the website Sleepyti.me. Try this handy sleep cycle calculator to help you create a snooze routine.

Bueller? Bueller? (Find Your Routine!)

A regular routine is crucial to creating a healthy lifestyle. Attending your classes helps you to establish your routine. As part of the Dolce Diet Principles, you'll be eating every 2-4 hours. Knowing the days and times of your classes will help you build out your meal schedule. Academically, it's important you show up – the same goes for your eating schedule. Whether you skip classes or skip meals, the end result will be: #FAIL

Franken-foods (Eat Earth-Grown Nutrients!)

Anything served with greasy plastic gloves and a hairnet terrifies me. Just forget about eating "food" that someone passes to you through a window. College tends to put you into situations where you need food quickly, and at odd hours – but now you can be prepared with some easy options from this book. The number one rule to follow is eat only earth-grown nutrients. If you simply stick to this one rule, no matter the situation, you will always choose correctly.

Liquid Fat (Drink More Water!)

Social drinking is a normal occurrence at college, and almost everyone does it. Here are a couple of things to remember. First, no amount of alcohol is good for you. It's a toxin – the reason it makes you feel drunk is because it's disrupting signals to your brain. Second, be intelligent: Moderate your intake, and only drink occasionally. If you drink until you puke, your body is telling you that you're an asshole. Don't be an asshole.

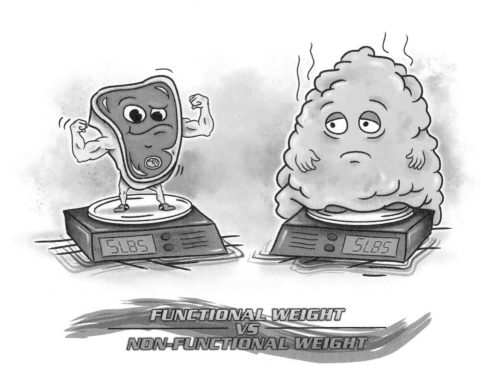

ARE YOU MADE OF JUNK?

"What you eat in private will show up in public."
~Rich 'Ace' Franklin

No matter how you phrase it, the idea of "you are what you eat" is the gospel of the human diet. How we feel, perform and look are the catalysts behind how we live our lives.

Just like a car won't perform well if you put vodka in its gas tank, neither will you. If you want to meet any physical challenge that life throws at you, from rushing a mile to class across a hilly campus without breaking a sweat, to competing as a varsity-level athlete, or shagging like Ron Jeremy (but with abs!), you need to give your body premium fuel.
Eating food is how your body replenishes itself. But what happens if your diet doesn't give your body the building blocks it needs? What if you give it sticks of dynamite instead? Yikes!

But what if you eat consciously and provide your body with all of the proper building blocks? It will function as it should, like a well-oiled machine. Every cell in your body will be running at full capacity. Your muscles will work better and tire less quickly, your organs will do their jobs more efficiently, while your blood delivers all of the nutrients they need, and your mind will be clear, with all the pistons firing as they should.

We are all capable of doing incredible things with our bodies! Whether your goal is athletic performance, gaining muscle mass, or losing weight to feel better in day-to-day life, making sure that your body is made of the right stuff is the most important step toward your goal.

You can stay alive by eating greasy double-bacon-cheeseburgers with fries – but not for long. On the other hand, you can eat to live, and have a long, vibrant life by sticking to clean, unprocessed foods. As a college student, now is the time to decide which lifestyle you'll pursue. It lays the foundation for Future You! And it doesn't take a college degree to figure out what Future You would prefer!

This is the time when you set your intellectual goals and work habits in stone. It is also the time when your body reaches full maturity, your metabolism begins to slow down, and your body begins to feel the effects of age.

You often see athletes reach their full potential at a young age, and then break down soon thereafter. This is because many merely focus on only muscles, eat poorly, and neglect their internal organs. But keeping your liver and kidneys healthy keeps toxins out of your blood. When your stomach and intestines are fed right, they can put food to work faster and more efficiently. If you eat foods that help your heart, it will keep everything running smoothly, increase your longevity and fortify your cognitive function. Yes, you must TRAIN YOUR BRAIN!

SHITTY PEOPLE

(THEY SUCK)

In Living Lean, we call these negative people who try to sway you from your path to lifestyle enlightenment CRABS IN THE POT. These people could be your so-called friends who make fun of you for not drinking to the point of crapping your pants or vomiting so hard you blow out your pupils (because that's always attractive in the light of day) or these crabs can be your family or your significant other. It's unfortunate, but true.

Don't be pulled down by others who might make fun of you (or get angry at you) for making positive changes in your life. These folks likely don't mean to sink their self-loathing claws into your sensitive skin. Often, they don't realize how negative they are, nor do they understand the effect their douche-baggery can have on you. TELL THEM! And then move on. We must lead by example, and hopefully, by seeing your positivity and progress, the Shitty People will follow in your footsteps.

An example of Crabs in the Pot Syndrome came in an email from Carlos. He recently graduated college, but it was a close call. His lack of preparedness and new sense of freedom had him running a bit wild. But one night, everything changed.

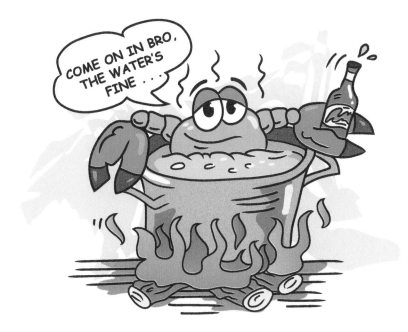

CARLOS

Age: 24 · **Starting Weight:** 191· **Current Weight:** 140

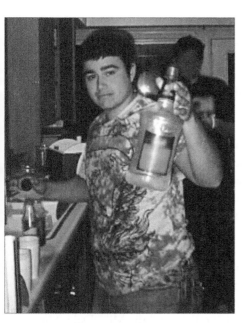
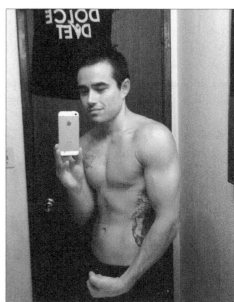

I started attending the University of Nevada Reno in fall 2007. I remember it was the first taste of freedom from my parents and I was ready to experience college. My parents helped me move into my dorm room and we said our goodbyes. Looking back at this moment, I knew that I was not ready to attend college. I did not have a focus or goal of what I wanted to do with my life. Like many other college students, I turned to partying, which led to a lot of binge drinking. My first semester, I drank almost every day and ate most of my meals in the dining hall. The dining hall basically consisted of pizza, burgers, sandwiches and more junk food. Most of my friends and peers ate all of the food and I never thought anything of it at the time. I found myself three years later weighing in at 191 lbs., and I'm only 5'7". My GPA was in the gutter, at only a 1.9. My binge drinking was out of control because I didn't know what I wanted to do with my life, and I was running away from what I could not fix. I fell into a slight depression and, like many other people, I used food for comfort.

Some nights I would drive through Jack in the Box and then drive next door to get some Taco Bell as well. After a night of partying my junior year, I woke up out of a blackout and couldn't stop puking. My whole body was numb and I was sweating like crazy and vomiting uncontrollably. I told myself that day that I wanted to change, and I couldn't do this anymore. I was so upset at myself that I was basically ready to drop out of college. I felt like a failure that day.

17

I woke up the next day and decided that this was going to be the start of something new. I started listening to the Joe Rogan podcast, and that's when I heard Mike Dolce for the first time. I bought Mike's books: Living Lean and 3 Weeks to Shredded. When the weekend came around, my friends brought home a case of beer like usual and asked me if I was ready to drink. I remember telling them that I was good on drinking for the night. For the next 8 months, I received huge amounts of peer pressure. It was unbelievable. People would make fun of me because I was on a diet, and no one around me really understood.

To stay busy and focused, I began training Brazilian Jiu Jitsu, and this changed my life forever. My goals became more strict, and I couldn't have been happier. I became really motivated when I started to see some changes in my body. At one point I had to go to the DMV and get a new picture because people didn't think it was my license. This really had me motivated, and nothing was going to stop me.

If there is any advice I can give, it's that you have to make the decision for yourself. You are going to encounter many obstacles and a lot of peer pressure, but that is all part of the journey. Like Mike says, you have to stay accountable. If you are just starting your college career, be very careful of who your friends are. There is nothing wrong with partying, but everything in moderation is key. Be careful of all the food around you and follow the principles. You can be on The Dolce Diet and still have a blast throughout college.

I am proud to say that I graduated recently from the university with a degree in General Studies. I barely squeezed by in school, and I never really found my passion until now. I can honestly say that diet and lifestyle are my passions now, and I love helping others out with the knowledge I have obtained from Living Lean and the Mike Dolce Show podcast. I now weigh 145 lbs. I went from a pant size of 36 to a size 30. I feel stronger than ever, and I can't wait to push myself even further.

Thank you so much, guys! You have changed my life forever, and I finally know what I want to do with my life: Help others through nutrition and guidance.

I DUB THEE, WORTHY!

"Sometimes the hardest part of the journey is believing you're worthy of the trip." ~ *Glenn Beck, The Christmas Sweater*

I don't know about you, but I don't put much stock in what others think of my lifestyle. I live my life my way, like Sinatra but with less cigarettes. It's alright if others think my lifestyle is "not normal." Their opinion has nothing to do with my actions.

My purpose in life is valid, without validation.

I'm aware of my self-worth, and I don't need a family member, friend or perfect stranger who wrote a book <clears throat> to tell me what I already know. And what is that exactly? That I'm worth making positive choices! That my life is worth more than simply following along with a pack of cows marching to their deaths around me.

Convenience and marketing has decomposed the way many of us view ourselves.

We've somehow forfeited the rich, succulent meals of old for the peel-the-plastic-off-and-zap-it quick-fix. The Gorton's Fisherman has replaced Father Time. We've rung our own bell and plummeted our stock.

Why are we resorting to so many fast foods? Do we actually have less time? No! We simply think less of it. If we valued our time, we'd value our choices.

Most meal plans fail because either 1) They are based on solid science but not sustainable or 2) They're full of shit.

What I'm giving you is the same set of principles my world-class athletes use to get in the best shape of their lives while juggling a schedule much busier than yours. Consider it a treasure map, where you each will find your own personal fortune. This lifestyle program produces immediate results. In fact, you've already changed by reading this far.

No longer will you go back to the old ways you once had. From the first meal, you will feel your energy rise. From the first week, your body will begin rapidly changing. From the first month, you will not believe you could eat what you once had.

Anybody can do this. Yes, I work with some of the most highly paid professionals in all of sports, but I also work with members of the lowest earning third-world cultures, where water itself is difficult to find.

These principles have proven effective everywhere...even the college campus. Now that you know the problem, allow me to share the solution.

THE SOLUTION

"Change your opinions, keep to your principles; change
your leaves, keep intact your roots."
~Victor Hugo

THE DOLCE DIET PRINCIPLES

(Don't panic. It's not really a diet.)

Every action you take is governed by a basic set of principles and guidelines. Whether you realize it or not, every decision you make springs forth from some idea you hold in your heart and mind. Usually, this is learned at home. Two-thirds of American adults will die of lifestyle related illness. These habits are reinforced by those around you. I'm sorry to say, guys, but two-thirds of you are learning how to get fat and die fast. We're also greatly influenced by our environmental surroundings, whether it's in the moment that you find yourself off-schedule and in an unfamiliar terrain forced to stop at a burrito shop or you've moved your entire life to a college campus and are taught to feed with the herd. When you function on autopilot, and simply act according to your habits and environment, you'll do what you've always done. If you want to make a change, you need to consciously adopt a new idea and focus on implementing it.

The fundamental dietary principles of my work are simple, but effective. They are sustainable on all continents within all cultures of any financial means. These basic guidelines will propel you to levels of health and fitness you've never considered, especially because it's so easy. Remember Sean?

 ## 1. Earth-Grown Nutrients

Up until the early 20th century, human diets were made up almost entirely of earth-grown nutrients. Our bodies have evolved and adapted over millions of years to digest natural foods and put them to work. The fewer steps it takes to bring a food out of the ground, field or stream, and into your mouth, the better. Our bodies have the tools to use these foods; they don't have the tools to use artificial ingredients made in laboratories. This may be a letdown, but you're not, in fact, a robot. Natural foods have this crazy ability to prevent you from feeling like a slug lodged in a pile of poop.

Remember, your body has a hard time digesting something it doesn't recognize. And just because you've been eating SpaghettiO's by the trough-full since you were 2 years old does not mean your body understands how to process them.

Difficult digestion is not the only reason to avoid chemically enhanced foods. They may have negative effects on your chemical make-up. One of the areas scientists are studying right now is the concept of epigenetics; how all this artificial processed goop could potentially change our DNA for generations to come. I don't know about you, but any food powerful enough to potentially give my great, great grandkid three eyes and a fin is a food not likely to grace my table.

If all you ate were earth-grown nutrients, harvested in their natural form in their natural habitat and consumed soon after they were picked, I guarantee that you would look and feel absolutely amazing! Think about it. Earth-grown nutrients have sustained all of life on this planet since the dawn of time. Our species and every other species in existence has thrived only because of earth-grown nutrients. Somewhere in the last 50-100 years a rich guy in a business suit sat down with a smart guy in a lab coat and they figured out a way to make money. They were going to control your health.

They were going to tell you what to eat based upon profit margins.
They were going to tell you where to eat by seducing your reptilian brain.
They were going to tell you how to eat by whispering "recommended guidelines" through the megaphone of government agencies.

These same entities are the ones forcing you to pay $6,000 a year to eat their highly processed, nutrient diminished, genetically modified Franken-foods. The average college campus cafeteria, though displayed differently, utilizes many of the same bulk ingredients as federal prisons. BOOM!

 ## 2. Eat Every 2-4 Hours Based Upon What You Just Did, And What You're About To Do

Your body is a machine. Much like a train, you must always add coal to the furnace to ensure the train keeps moving. Too much coal and you will snuff out the fire, too little and the train won't have the energy to continue traveling. Your body mirrors this principle in that it must always be well nourished in order to function properly at all times. As a result, one should eat every 2-4 hours based upon current activity levels AND your projected activities for the rest of the day. This will ensure that your metabolism is constantly moving and your body has the tools necessary to not only sustain life, but to continually grow and improve.

If you have the day off and you're relaxing around the dorm, you should not be eating excessive calories that we now know will slow down our metabolism and rob our energy.

On these days, eat lighter and more often instead. (You'll see the recipes later in this book.) On days when you're carrying a heavy course load and you're still sneaking in your workouts and keeping an active social life, we look for more nutrient-dense foods to supply us with the energy to sustain such a pace.

3. Eat Until Satisfied, Not Until Full

The typical overweight, undersexed waste of college space often eats huge meals and stuffs their face until they're so full that they can barely move. Not good for the metabolism. In fact, while your body desperately tries to break down this massive meal, it must pull resources from other areas of your body, making you extremely lethargic and over-stressing the digestive system.

You know what I'm talking about because you've felt it. It's disgusting. How many of you have eaten a huge Italian meal and three days later it's still trying to make its way out!? Gross!

What's the rush? Why must you eat two days worth of calories in one sitting? Is it worth it? Is it worth feeling slow and sluggish and flatulent? Do you like looking down to see the top of your beer belly and nothing else? Why not eat moderate sized meals often, speeding up your metabolism, sustaining a high energy output, allowing your digestive system to rapidly absorb and process the nutrients, keeping you strong and fit and virile? Trust me, it's much better eating six meals a day than eating one very tasty but slow-digesting slop fest – especially when you wake up with abs the next morning. As a rule of thumb, I always want to feel as if I could go for a 30 minute jog after any meal, not my hardest pace, not even a fast pace, but when I push myself away from the table, I still feel light and fit enough to do anything.

Let your digestion be your diet coach. It will tell you immediately if you've messed up and applaud you for choosing correctly! Eating should be a pleasurable, happy experience – not a journey between two states of discontent.

 ## 4. Don't Count Calories, Make Calories Count!

One of the biggest misconceptions in the weight-loss world by far is that calories are the panacea of weight-loss gold. Again, friends, I implore you! Please hear me! Calorie counting is bullshit! If calorie counting worked, you all would look like me; so would your parents and their coworkers and everybody else you know. Ask anyone about their diet and they immediately start talking about their calories. I've said it before and I'll say it again: Don't count calories! Make calories count!

Your body doesn't simply run on calories. Let's say the average donut has 400 calories. A well-balanced lunch of 400 calories can also be brown rice, wild-caught salmon and grilled asparagus. I'm currently 195 lbs. at 6 percent body fat. If the calorie myth were true, I'd look exactly the same if I ate donuts for every meal.

The more nutrient dense your food, the better you feel regardless of calories. A 500 calorie fast food cheeseburger isn't as healthy as 500 calories of spinach. Many people eat two or three or even four cheeseburgers in a single meal to get full. How many of you can eat 70 cups of spinach in one sitting, which equals just one of those cheeseburgers, at nearly 500 calories? There's also approximately 70 grams of protein in that same amount of spinach, by the way.

When my athletes are in the midst of a 20-40 lb. weight cut, they do so in the healthiest manner possible by maintaining the utmost nutrient density of each precious calorie they consume. There is no room for excess in that situation. And the principle applies to everyone.

Guys, would you rather invite your buddy and four thirsty dudes to your party or that same buddy and four smokin' hot girls? Like I said, don't focus on the quantity, focus on the quality as it pertains to your goal.

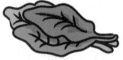 ## 5. Be Accountable

I wrote this book for you, but I can't do it for you. It has to come from within. Just the action of reading to this point shows you have it within you to make a change. The best part about The Dolce Diet is that it's so easy to implement into any lifestyle, especially yours! We start by making simple choices each day, each meal, each morning, and we allow those choices to gain momentum.

The most common statement about our program is "It is not a diet, it's a lifestyle." Success is also a lifestyle. Bill Gates, Will Smith, Richard Branson, Duane "The Rock" Johnson, and so many more all have this one characteristic in common. They are accountable. They accept projects based on deadlines, wake up early, perform their work and also take the time to be accountable to their own health. Any of you with an entrepreneurial mind must realize immediately the first challenge you must overcome is managing yourself. Once you can do that, you can do anything. If you cannot control what you consume, I'm sorry, you won't be able to control anything as life becomes more complex. Now is the time, today is the day, the very next choice you make will be in your best interest. As will the next one and the next one and the next one. And in this way we become better every day. Even just one tiny percent better is BETTER! Aren't you worth "better?" I say YES!

GOAL SETTING
& ACTION STEPS

"I know where I'm going and I know the truth, and I don't have to be what you want me to be. I'm free to be what I want." *~Muhammad Ali*

Without goals, what is our purpose? Goals help keep us accountable. Goals are the fuel in the machine of life.

Just the word GOAL invokes a destination. Whether it be an end zone, a mountain top or a smaller dress size, we all know what a goal should be. The problem I often come across is that people have loose goals. They kid themselves by pretending to have set a goal, when really they just have a wish.

"I want to lose weight," is the most common wish, but it often goes no further than that statement. When confronted with this person I always ask, "How much weight do you want to lose? What deadline have you set? Let me see your action steps to get there." Guess what the most common answer to my questions is: a blank stare.

This is when I switch into coach mode and make sure my friend has a clear plan and walks away with a newfound purpose. Now it's your turn. Here are three steps to setting goals:

STEP 1 • BE SPECIFIC
"I WILL (not want to) lose 40 lbs."
Now you have a very clear picture of your exact destination.
There is no confusion here.

STEP 2 • SET A DEADLINE
"I WILL lose 40 lbs. in 120 days."
Now you have a specific timeline. No more circling the drain, waiting to begin.
The clock is now ticking.

STEP 3 • COMMIT THROUGH ACTION STEPS
"I WILL lose 40 lbs. in 120 days by following these ACTION STEPS."

ACTION STEP 1 – Read up on the Dolce Diet Principles in this book and create my own lifestyle approach to healthy living using the philosophy, recipes and exercise programs that Mike has already laid out, focusing on those most suited to my own ability, goals and medical history.

ACTION STEP 2 – Be consistent. For the next 120 days (and rest of my life), I will dedicate myself to achieving this goal and hold myself 100 percent accountable. Regardless of what unexpected trial or tribulation may come up in my life, I will continue on with my goal until I have found success.

ACTION STEP 3 – Create a support system. This may be your family, friends, team, coworkers or online community. I have started such a community at **MYDolceDiet.com** for all of us to support, motivate and inspire each other as we collectively travel toward our own unique goals. Pro-athletes, bikini models, lawyers, students, moms, dads, law enforcement professionals and many others from all walks of life are members, and the community is thriving!

ACTION STEP 4 – Begin TODAY! There is no better time than the present. Don't push it off until Monday. Start now, as best you can, and continue making improvements the first few days. It doesn't matter if you haven't gone grocery shopping yet, or have a class in 15 minutes. Begin moving toward your goal immediately and constantly work to improve your situation as you go. Flip that switch in your brain and start NOW!

The Action Steps above are general but apply to each of you. I also instruct my students to sit down at a quiet table with a notebook they have purchased specifically for the purpose of goal setting and write down everything. Jot down your goals, a more complete version of these action steps with greater detail as it relates to your specific situation, your daily body weight, progress with your workouts, frustrations, successes and so on. This book becomes your training partner, support system, cherished friend and annoying cheerleader, reminding you of how far you have come.

What do you want to look like 6 months from now? A year? What about 5 years? Most people aren't forward thinking enough to plan what they'll have for lunch today, and they certainly aren't thinking about what type of body and physique they want to have 5 years from now, but they should. Forward thinking will allow you to make better choices today. Future You will thank you for not saddling yourself with a monster-truck spare tire, flabby arms, cottage-cheese butt or man-boobs.

Remember our friend, Carlos, who is now 51 lbs. lighter? Yes, he scared himself shit-less, a condition widely known to be a great catalyst of change, but hopefully, you don't need to go to the Dark and Scary Place to find motivation. Carlos figured out what he wanted, physically and mentally, and he attacked his goals despite what his friends were doing around him, despite living away at college, and despite all the forces of the universe being stacked against him. He made a choice. And you can, too. Ultimately, you know everything I have said above. Getting you to be accountable and motivating you to start today was MY goal! Now it's time to define your own!

EDWIN

Age: 23 · **Starting Weight:** 189 · **Current Weight:** 174

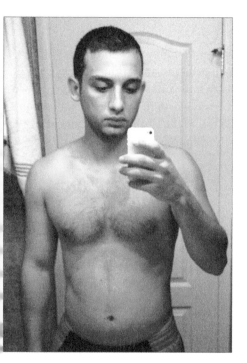 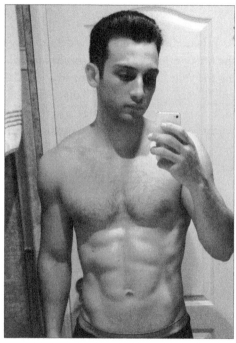

I was always active and played sports throughout my life. But everything changed once I stopped exercising and began eating extremely unhealthy foods. It all started when my health reached an ultimate low one year ago. I had gained about 15 lbs. and looked like a very unhealthy young man.

During this time, I was diagnosed with Crohn's Disease, a chronic inflammatory disease of the intestines. I was miserable and in excruciating pain. I couldn't believe how my life had been turned upside down. I beat myself up for a few months, feeling sorry for myself.

This is when I decided to follow Mike Dolce's principles. I bought Living Lean and Living Lean Cookbook, read them, and they lit a fire inside of me. I was ready to change my life! I got in the kitchen and followed Mike's recipes to a healthier life. I became fascinated with Mike's philosophies and fell in love with his food (especially the Breakfast Bowl!). At the same time I began following The Dolce Diet, I joined a local gym. I put together a one-two punch that dramatically changed my life. My symptoms began to slowly go away! I never felt better and I couldn't believe it.

The lifestyle that Mike taught me has kept my chronic illness to an absolute minimum. This is why I will never go back to my old ways.
Mike Dolce changed my life. He gave me the spark that has now lit an enormous fire. I now exercise six days a week, and follow Mike's Living Lean philosophies/recipes. Mike impacted my life so drastically that I am back at college studying kinesiology and seeking a career in the health and fitness world. BOOM!

* * *

As Edwin discovered, our insides are very real. Even though you're young and living the life of a college student, health and disease do exist and are lurking about just waiting for your lifestyle decisions to allow them entry into your situation. Luckily, Edwin saw the signs and made a change. He decided he was worth it. We must all allow our inner cogs, wheels and widgets to operate at the top of their game so we can consistently be at the top of ours. Look in the mirror and simply know you're worth the better things in life. Flip the switch.

THE TOTALLY NOT BORING
CHAPTER ON HABITS

"We are what we repeatedly do.
Excellence, then, is not an act, but a habit." ~*Aristotle*

I never understood New Year's resolutions; why people wait until January 1 to make a compelling lifestyle change. Consider this: You are so sick and disgusted and disappointed and disillusioned at this moment that as of the beginning of the NEXT year you're FINALLY going to flip the switch and make a change. WHAT?! Does that make sense? Why not start NOW?

Resolutions are merely statements that bear no consequence without action. Actions are the process of predictable habits. To be successful, we simply create a set of habits for you to follow throughout your day that easily improves your life and general well-being.

Today is your January 1. It's New YOU Day!

Research has shown that it takes 21 days to form a habit. That's not long at all! If you're consistent, there's no reason your new, healthier habits can't become a reality. Try making your own habit chart! Be honest with yourself. No one needs to see this list but you! Jot down all the habits you want to change and a simple way to axe them over time. Now you're on a mission!

Habit Chart

The following are examples of habits to break, habits to create and the action steps to get you there.

HABIT TO KICK ★	NEW HABIT ★	ACTION STEP
No more soda, beer, processed juices or energy drinks!	More water, green tea, raw smoothies, and black coffee!	Drink one less "bad habit" drink every day, replacing each with a "new habit" drink until I'm totally off all the crap!
Vending machine food, fast food, convenience store crap.	Stock up on bulk almonds, cashews, raisins, figs, chia seeds and hemp seeds.	Plan my meals for the next three days and shop for them!
Watch too much TV, smoke too much weed, don't exercise.	Smoke weed outside and bring a Frisbee.	Buy a Frisbee!

Of all bad habits, and there are many, the most important one to kick is procrastination. Fortunately for you, I'm an expert at defeating deferment. I have to be! The professional fighter that gets punched, kicked, bent, twisted and slammed twice a day, six days a week has more than enough reasons to put off today's training until tomorrow. The key to beating procrastination is staying accountable. We must be accountable to ourselves.

Your percentage for success dramatically increases by adhering to these three simple rules:

- **Rule 1.** Set a goal.
- **Rule 2.** Set a date.
- **Rule 3.** Set your action plan.

The rest of this book will give you your action plan.

THE ACTION

"When it is obvious that the goals cannot be reached,
don't adjust the goals, adjust the action steps." *~Confucius*

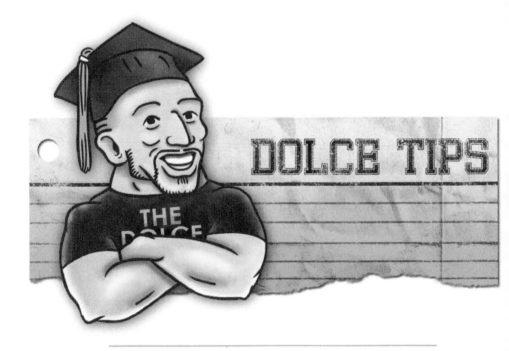

DOLCE TIPS

TIP: *Keep your kitchen supplies in a box under your bed or in your closet. Wash them immediately and bring them right back. I learned this technique when I was on Season 7 of The Ultimate Fighter living in a four-bedroom home with 16 dudes.*
Kind of like Lord of The Flies with cage fighters.

HOW TO EAT WELL IN ALL CAMPUS LIVING SITUATIONS

Many of you will have some version of a college meal plan associated with your campus cafeteria or dining hall. All of you should look to this menu to supplement your own nutritional lifestyle, not the other way around.

When I travel, I always bring in my backpack many of the very same foods you'll find on the grocery list at the end of this book. I would prefer to have a backpack full of food with barely enough room for socks and underwear than three suitcases filled with my entire wardrobe. Like Pac-man races around for his pellets, I'm always on the look-out for fresh earth-grown nutrients and purified water sources.

When you walk into a cafeteria, ask yourself: Which of these foods is on my grocery list? What can I stock up on and supply my room with? What are the freshest and most natural items on today's menu?

Eat those items and those items only. Stuff your backpack to stock up your room. Get your money's worth!

Below are some inexpensive and easy-to-find mainstays that will make your college life either a-la Hugh Hefner or Honey Boo-Boo. You choose!

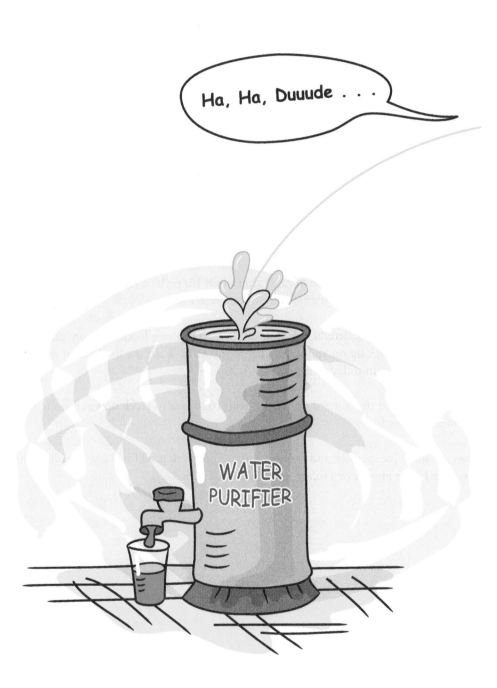

COLLEGE ESSENTIALS LIST

Go through these lists and see how many products you can bring to your dorm, suite or apartment. Ask your parents and friends to buy them for you online and have them delivered to your school address to save you the cost. Check out **CollegeDietGuide.com** for links to many of these Dolce Approved products at a discount.

EQUIPMENT

Filtered water pitcher (Brita, PUR, Berkey) – Get an inexpensive water filter that is built into a pitcher like a Brita or PUR, or our favorite, Berkey. Top it off from the sink or water fountain. With the Berkey, you can actually pour your toilet water in there (just in case one of your asshole friends tries to do it, you'll be grossed out, but safe).

Electric tea kettle – From soothing teas to morning coffee to belly-filling oatmeal, a tea kettle is the Rosetta Stone that unlocks eating well in a restrictive dorm environment. You can find a good, inexpensive kettle online for under $15. You can hard boil eggs in a kettle as easily as you can in a pot!

Mini refrigerator – Having a refrigerator in your dorm room opens up your food choices. You can get a mini fridge for around $65 and a mini fridge-freezer combo unit for around $100. If you can get your hands on a used one, even better!

Blender – You can get a decent quality machine for about $20, though you may want to spend a bit more. A quality blender can be used to make fruit and vegetable smoothies, post-workout shakes, quick and healthy breakfasts on the go as well as mixed drinks for sexy time. Right, Hef?

Electric hot plate, Electric grill, Toaster oven, Slow-cooker – If your school allows these, great! Bring them along. You can use them to prepare or reheat a wide variety of dishes, and create your own mini-kitchen. If I had my choice of just one it would be a 15-inch electric skillet that you can easily unplug, dismantle and hide around your room in less than 30 seconds (like I do in hotel rooms before the maids come in).

KITCHENWARE
Note: All pots and pans should be stainless steel

1-quart pot
4-quart pot
8-quart pot (great if you have a kitchen and you REALLY like to cook!)
9-inch pan
12-inch pan
Spatula (stainless steel)
Large spoon (stainless steel)
Forks, Spoons, Knives (stainless steel)
Large pasta bowl
Small cereal bowl
Dinner plates
Mug
Water glass
Measuring cups
Measuring spoons
Cutting board
Strainer
Can opener

CLEANING
(Yes, you may be washing items in your bathroom sink. **Keep it clean!**)

Paper-towels
Napkins
Dish towel
Dish detergent
Scrub sponge
Anti-bacterial kitchen wipes
Drying mat

FOOD STORAGE

Glass containers with lids
Ziploc bags (or similar resealable bags)
Aluminum foil
Plastic wrap

Note: Whether you're plundering your dining hall for food to store in your dorm, or you want to preserve that Chia Pudding so it's ready for breakfast, our number one choice for food storage is glass containers with air-tight lids. Glass products are environmentally friendly, resistant to mold and bacteria, preserve the nutrient density of your food, and do not leach plastic toxins. One-gallon Ziploc bags are also the perfect way to store your cashew-and-raisin trail mix that you walk around campus with so you're never without a healthy meal option. There are many other easy water-proof, freezer-safe storage options. Find the ones that work best for your living situation.

MISCELLANEOUS

Hot/cold travel mug – Bring meals or beverages with you when you're in a hurry
Large storage bin – Safely stow your kitchenware

SAFELY NAVIGATING
THE COLLEGE CAFETERIA

Many students complain that they're sick of the campus food before their freshman year ends because they end up eating the same things a few times each week. Of that limited list, very few options would be healthy. Planning ahead and knowing what to look for can help you avoid the bad stuff.

Always look for vegetables and fruit of the freshest variety. We always want to find foods as close to their natural state as possible.

This includes:
FRESH
Apples
Asparagus
Avocado
Bananas
Berries
Broccoli
Carrots
Eggplant
Grapes
Kale
Nuts
Oranges
Raisins
Seeds
Spinach
Tomatoes

COOKED
Lean proteins (typically chicken or fish, but stay away from tuna salad as the mayonnaise and other additives devalue any benefit)
Extra virgin olive oil & balsamic vinegar (for salad dressing)

Of the cooked food options in a cafeteria, steamed, grilled, boiled and broiled are best, with no seasoning or sauces. Always ask for all toppings to be put on the side.

Cafeteria meat is daunting. Don't be afraid to ask the chef where the meat came from. You'd be hard pressed to find a locally grown, wild-caught hot dog.

Try to avoid dairy, especially on a college campus. Due to cost, the quality of cheese and milk (and bread too) on a campus is extremely low. After all, colleges are a business and they're likely buying in bulk to feed thousands of hungry students.

Sodas and fountain drinks must be avoided at all costs. The empty calories, artificial sugars, chemical contaminates and even the carbonation can dramatically disrupt your digestion and the functioning of your cells. Stick with water, fresh brewed teas and black coffee (to which I always add one teaspoon of coconut oil).

The lesson in all this? Know what you're eating and be accountable to your goals.

EATING FOR EXAM DAY

Eating for exam day starts weeks before the test. Your diet and health are like a ship – it takes a lot of energy, focus and time to turn it all the way around. If you're eating like crap the day before your exam, you won't be feeling your best, no matter what you eat. So, just like your schoolwork, don't leave your diet to the last minute.

When you're preparing and studying for an exam, make sure that you're even more diligent with your food plan and always remember to bring food with you. Nuts and raisins, an apple and peanut butter or a Caveman Foods snack bar, along with a bottle of water are items you never should be without. (CavemanFoods.com/Dolce)

The day of the test, make sure you're awake a few hours before the exam starts. It takes time for your brain to turn on and function at its full capacity.

Eat breakfast! Know the day before what you'll be eating so you can plan ahead. The Dolce Diet Breakfast Bowl is always a great option! (See recipe in the back of the book.) The last thing you want is to be sitting in your exam, and suddenly get hungry or thirsty while you're solving a complex math problem or writing an essay. Besides, no one wants to hear your stomach's rendition of Jurassic Park.

Complete meals with complex carbohydrates fortified with a high percentage of healthy fiber like Bob's Red Mill Oat Bran; essential fats from sources like hemp seeds and chia seeds, which slow digestion and allow for a long source of mind enhancing brain fuel; simple sugars in the form of fresh fruits and berries to give you that immediate perk and get your body moving; and finally, water – lots of it – to aid in ample digestion and ensure proper hydration during your sometimes marathon-esque test taking.

Why all this food? The act of thinking requires energy! Therefore, you need brain food! A well-fed brain can focus better for longer, which, in college, is crucial for achieving your goals. So what makes good brain food?

Stay super hydrated for an efficient metabolism and bring a coffee with a teaspoon of coconut oil in it to class to keep the synapses firing and your appetite satiated.

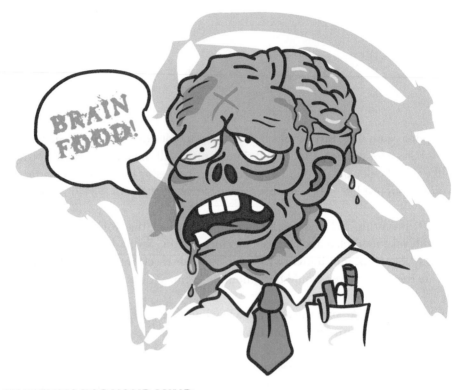

MUNCHIES FOR YOUR MIND

Antioxidants
Fruits like blueberries, strawberries, apples and red grapes will help keep your mind sharp with their natural sugars and immunity boosting antioxidants.

Whole Grains
Slow-digesting, energy-dense foods like oats, brown rice, buckwheat and quinoa are a key element in aiding mental agility. These foods have high fiber contents and can help us to feel fuller longer.

Omega-3 Fatty Acids
Salmon, tuna, beans, walnuts, flaxseeds and hemp seeds are your brain's best buds. Omega-3's have been widely researched and may stave off depression, fortify mental well-being and in a recent study, even increase functioning in the portion of the brain associated with happiness. :)

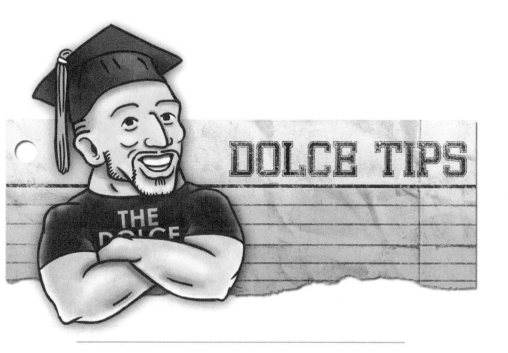

DOLCE TIPS

TIP: *Rinsing canned beans may leave you feeling less gassy after eating them! Why? Canned beans contain a sugar called oligosaccharide, which the human body is typically unable to digest. Once it hits the large intestine, the bacteria in the intestine feeds on the sugar and happily multiplies! Let's just say what happens next can be likened to The Big Bang! Always rinse your beans!*

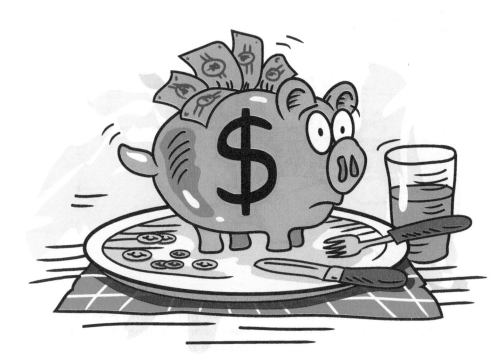

SHOP INTELLIGENTLY

"The best rosebush, after all, is not that which has the fewest thorns, but that which bears the finest roses." *~Henry Van Dyke*

The easiest way to stock your room is to simplify how you shop.

Two rules:
Never shop when you're hungry.
Make your grocery list based on meals you've already planned.

Do not buy your food wastefully. Remember what I say: Don't count calories, make calories count. And when you're spending your hard earned money – or your parents' – you better make sure you're getting the highest quality nutrition your money can buy.

Pop Tarts, ramen noodles and Mac N' Cheese are for fat little kids who grow up into fat, lonely virgins. I'm not joking. It's much better and cost efficient to buy dried goods jam-packed with nutrient-dense deliciousness that have a long shelf life like nuts, seeds, oats, grains, fruit and trusted snack bars like Dolce Approved Caveman Bars. Caveman Foods makes some of the most delicious and nutritious snack bars I have ever tasted. They have a growing product line and continue to push the boundaries of using the highest possible ingredients while maintaining excellent flavor. Website: **CavemanFoods.com/Dolce** (Use promo code **DOLCE** for a discount.)

My pantry is stuffed with cashews, almonds, peanuts, chia seeds, hemp seeds, sunflower seeds, pistachios, oat bran, quinoa, raisins, figs, dates and coconut flakes, in addition to dried beans, lentils and more exotic grains. I can live on these foods with a few servings of fresh fruits, vegetables and purified water procured throughout my day. All these ingredients are easily found at big box stores like Sam's Club and Wal-Mart, local mom and pop hippie health food stores, and internet retailers like Amazon.

Don't be shy when it comes to your health and wellness. Offset your costs by making it clear to people who give you gifts that you want gift cards to stores such as these for food. You might be surprised at how generous your loved ones are if they don't think you're going to spend it on weed and beer pong.

I strongly suggest you do your major grocery shopping one day per week earlier in the day when you have the least amount to do, and then approximately three days later make a quick store run to stock up on fresh fruit and perishable items.

A good rule of thumb is to purchase only what you've planned meals for. You don't want to buy a few pounds of tomatoes just because they're on sale, then end up throwing them out because they've gone bad before you can eat them.

It sounds silly but the average American throws away up to 40 percent of the food they purchase. Besides, it's better to go to the store a few times each week for your produce. That way you're always eating fresh food.

Always have a budget. ALWAYS. This is one of the essential habits that must be implemented into your life. Remember Sean? His parents were spending $3,000 a semester that he was able to shave down to just $800 in that same amount of time when given a budget of just $1,000. I'm pretty sure Sean didn't tell his parents where the extra $200 went.

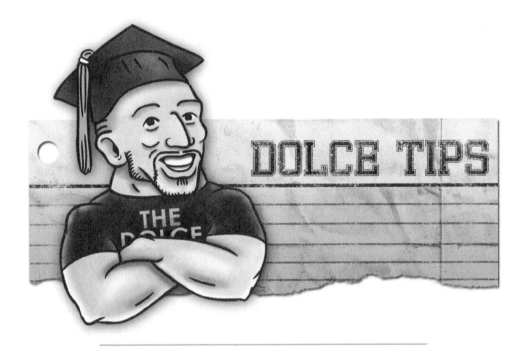

Tip: Always keep these five questions in mind when you shop:

What will I use it for, and when?
How much does it cost per unit? (Hint: This is typically found on the lower lefthand corner of the shelf tag.)
Can I get a better deal on something similar?
Where can I store it, and for how long?
How versatile is this ingredient; can I use it in several recipes?

DOLCE APPROVED EARTH-GROWN SUPPLEMENT LIST

This list contains products you may not be accustomed to using in your everyday life, but you should!

GREEN TEA

There are three predominant types of tea: green, black and oolong. Green tea is the least processed and provides the most antioxidant polyphenols, notably a catechin called epigallocatechin-3-gallate (EGCG), which researchers believe to be responsible for most of its health benefits. Green tea contains three major components that have been shown to promote fat loss: catechins, caffeine and theanine.

In a 2004 study in which mice were fed diets containing 2 percent green tea powder for 16 weeks, visceral fat decreased by 76.8 percent in those receiving green tea compared to the control group. Green tea also decreased blood levels of triglycerides (the chemical form in which most fats exist in the body).

Green tea also appears to increase endurance, allowing you to train harder and exercise longer, as the catechins appear to stimulate the use of fatty acids by the liver and muscle cells. This ability to burn fat more efficiently offers a reduction in reliance on glycogen — stored energy in the muscles from carbohydrate rich food sources. This mechanism is believed to contribute in reduction in body fat and overall increase in muscular tone and fitness.

Lastly, green tea is delicious, very inexpensive and extremely easy to implement in any college situation.

DANDELION

As far as all-natural diuretics go, Dandelion is hands down my favorite. We have proven its merit with my athletes during their pre-competition weight cuts.
As with all things, I do prefer to get real dandelion leaves and roots from my local grocery store to mix into salads and teas, but also leave the option open to try any reputable brand in bottled form for your convenience.

On their website, the University Of Maryland Medical Center states, "Traditionally, dandelion has been used as a diuretic to increase the amount of urine in order to get rid of too much fluid." This could be a great option to naturally reduce some of that post-party bloating or pre-menstrual swelling, or to tighten up for a trip to the beach!

COFFEE

I'm a fan of coffee. There, I said it! I'm assuming that you also are in the 54 percent majority of adults in the U.S. who would be considered a habitual coffee drinker, according to the National Coffee Association.

In fact, it is stated that 146 billion cups of coffee are consumed in the U.S. each year, nearly three times that of tea! Now, I'm not in that group, as I typically consume green tea to coffee in the opposite 3:1 ratio.

That being said, coffee can be a great thermogenic aid, assisting some in fat loss and a nice cognitive perk before a big test or an intense workout. The major downfall with most cups of coffee may not be the caffeine, as much as it is all the artificial sweeteners and creamers many of you add. If you truly want to go FULL DOLCE and achieve that slim, sexy and smart body you deserve, try adding just 1 teaspoon of coconut oil in your coffee to add fat-burning, mind-enhancing, hunger-eliminating essential fats that offer a creaminess similar to a dairy product with none of the guilt!

CHIA SEEDS

The word CHIA comes from an ancient Mayan translation meaning STRENGTH. Just like our ancient brethren learned over 5,000 years ago, chia seeds are a super food offering a sustained source of strength for any of us smart enough to mix them into our own modern life.

The ancient Mayans would carry them in satchels on their backs or around their waists as they ventured off on long hunting trips or war parties, where they would need a sustainable source of energy, while not being weighed down with their own traditional cooking implements.

Chia packs 3 grams of protein, 5 grams of carbohydrates, 5 grams of fiber and 4.5 grams of essential fats per tablespoon. In fact, chia seeds contain more health-boosting Omega-3 essential fats than an equal portion of salmon!

Absorbing up to 12 times its own weight, chia seeds expand, creating a feeling of satisfaction after consuming, and curbing those nasty hunger pains that may lead you to less healthy options. My athletes and I regularly add a teaspoon of chia seeds to each 16 ounces of water we drink to keep our energy high, our metabolism moving and our muscles strong, just like the ancient warriors!

HEMP SEEDS

Personally, hemp seeds are my favorite source of protein, far besting most popular sports performance products on the market. Sorry to say that you will not get a buzz after ingesting any of the regulated, quality hemp products on the market, but you must make sure your brand is reputable and seek the guidance of any governing body you may have to answer to. **CollegeDietGuide.com** offers Dolce Approved hemp seed options.

That being said, most of my athletes and myself enjoy hemp seeds as a part of our healthy daily meal plan, and the results speak for themselves. Hemp seeds are a great way to get an ideal ratio of Omega-6 to Omega-3, including the rare essential fatty acid known as Gamma-Linolenic Acid (GLA), as well as 5 grams of protein per 2 tablespoons! Plus, they are delicious!

This list is constantly changing! As science rapidly expands, so does our list. Please refer to **CollegeDietGuide.com** for a list of Dolce Approved supplements that will take you to the next level.

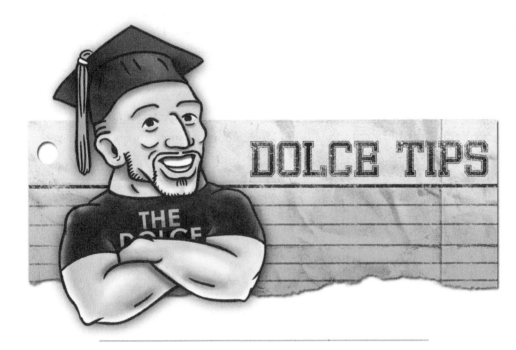

TIP: *Never go hungry! Always have some sort of healthy snack in your backpack! Here are some of my favorites:*

- *Dried fruits like raisins or banana chips*
- *Fruits with a tough skin like apples or oranges*
- *Nuts like cashews or almonds*
- *Caveman Bars*
- *Peanut butter or almond butter*
- *Always, always, always have WATER! Often when we think we're hungry, we're really just thirsty!*

DOLCE APPROVED GROCERY LIST

To the best of your budget and geographic availability, always choose wild-caught, free-range, naturally fed, humanely procured non GMO (genetically modified) organic and local ingredients.

Whew! That was a mouthful!

I'm sure I could get even more specific with this list but you get the picture.

Dolce Diet Principle #1 - Eating earth-grown nutrients is the most important point in this book. The common misconception is that eating healthy is expensive, typically because an organic chicken breast is $6, while the conventional chemical creation packaged and processed with sodium and pumped full of fluid to increase weight is $3. The amount of nutrition each provides and your body in turn absorbs is of no comparison. The more nutrient dense your foods, the less food you need to eat to satisfy your hunger and fuel your metabolism.

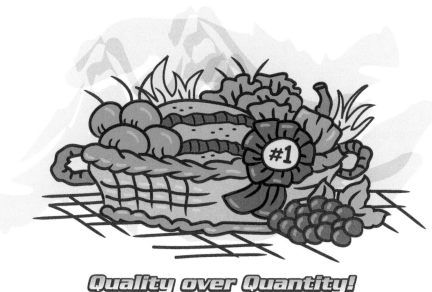

Quality over Quantity!

Note: Our first choice should always be wild-caught products. However, the complexity of your college living situation might not allow you to use such ingredients. In these cases, high quality canned or vacuum-packed lean proteins, dried fruits and other similarly packed products are great alternatives. In my home, we stock up on canned, wild-caught sockeye salmon. We don't eat it every day but it is always there when we need it and a much better alternative to most restaurant bought items. It's nice to have some of these products on your shelf when bad weather strikes or the zombies come knocking.

FRUIT
Apples
Avocados
Bananas
Blueberries
Dates
Figs
Grapes
Oranges
Raisins
Strawberries

VEGETABLES
Asparagus
Baby spinach
Broccoli
Brussels sprouts
Carrots
Celery
Chard
Cucumber
Eggplant
Green peppers
Kale
Onions
Red peppers
Sweet potatoes
Tomatoes

GRAINS
Buckwheat
Brown rice
Oat bran
Pasta (brown rice)
Quinoa
Sprouted grain breads & wraps
Whole grain bread & wraps

NUTS
Almonds
Cashews
Nut butters (peanut, almond, cashew, hazelnut)
Pistachios
Pecans
Walnuts

SEEDS
Chia seeds
Flaxseeds
Hemp seeds
Sunflower seeds

LEGUMES
Black beans
Garbanzo beans
Kidney beans
Lentils
Pinto beans
Red beans

OILS
Coconut oil (Very diverse: great for cooking, adding to coffee and tea, and a great moisturizer)
Extra virgin olive oil (for dressing)
Grapeseed oil (for cooking)
Hemp oil (great in smoothies)
Peanut oil (for cooking)

DAIRY/NON-DAIRY ALTERNATIVE
Almond milk
Coconut milk
Cottage cheese
Goat cheese
Greek yogurt
Hemp milk
Vegenaise

ANIMAL PROTEIN

Bison
Buffalo
Eggs
Elk
Poultry
Salmon
Tuna

BEVERAGES

Coconut water
Coffee
Green tea (the kind you brew via a tea bag or loose leaves)
Water

OTHER ITEMS

Agave
Balsamic vinegar
Black olives
Coconut (shredded, unsweetened)
Dill pickle relish (unsweetened)
Honey
Horseradish
Ketchup
Mustard

SPICES

Basil
Black pepper
Cayenne pepper
Cinnamon
Garlic
Oregano
Paprika
Parsley
Sea salt
Thyme

Note: This shopping list can be printed at **CollegeDietGuide.com.**

DORM-FRIENDLY RECIPES

Many of these recipes are built around low-cost groceries and ease of preparation, and are designed for college students who don't have much time or money. None of the recipes we've included here require a rice cooker, pot or pan, however, if you're able to have these items in your dorm you will be able to prepare a wider variety of meals, especially those in The Dolce Diet: Living Lean Cookbook that involve pasta and quinoa. For now, our goal is to arm you with some basic, yet delicious recipes.

★ BREAKFAST ★

Breakfast Bowl
Equipment: Tea kettle

Ingredients
1/2 cup oat bran or buckwheat* (*Gluten-free)
1/4 cup raisins
1/2 cup berries
1/2 sliced banana
1 Tbsp. all-natural nut butter
1 Tbsp. chia seeds
1 pinch cinnamon
1 cup water
dash of almond milk (optional)

Directions
In a tea kettle, bring 1 cup water to boil and add to bowl.
Mix in oat bran, stirring often until desired consistency is reached.
Mix in chia seeds, raisins and cinnamon.
Add in nut butter and top with banana.
Add in a dash of almond milk or water to thin out oat bran if desired.

Granola Berry Smash
Equipment: None

Ingredients
1/4 cup blueberries
1/4 cup strawberries
1/4 cup granola
1/4 cup almond milk
dash of cinnamon

Directions
Add berries to bowl.
Top with granola and almond milk.
Sprinkle with cinnamon.

Oats & Dates Bowl
Equipment: Tea kettle

Ingredients
1/4 cup oat bran
2 Tbsp. hemp seeds
2 Tbsp. chia seeds
3/4 cup water, boiled
splash of almond milk (optional)
dash of cinnamon
1/4 cup chopped dates (can substitute with raisins!)

Directions
Bring water to a boil in tea kettle.
Add oats, dates, seeds, and dash of cinnamon to bowl and cover with small plate.
Let sit about 10 minutes to thicken.
Add splash of almond milk and mix well.

Eggs & Avocado Bowl
Equipment: Tea kettle

Ingredients
2 eggs
1/2 avocado
1/4 cup brown lentils
pinch of Himalayan sea salt
pepper, to taste
3 cups water

Directions
To hard-boil eggs: Place eggs in tea kettle with water and bring to a boil. Let eggs sit in kettle about 12 minutes after the kettle shuts off.

Remove eggs and run cold water over egg shell for 1 minute.

Tap egg on hard surface to crack it, and then peel the shell.

Add eggs to a bowl with the avocado.

Sprinkle salt and pepper, mix and serve.

Egg Salad Sandwich
Equipment: Tea kettle

Ingredients
  2 whole eggs, hard-boiled, peeled and chopped
  1/4 onion, chopped
  1 tsp. mustard
  dash of Himalayan sea salt
  dash of black pepper
  1/2 avocado
  3 cups water
  whole grain or sprouted grain bread/wrap

Directions
Place eggs in tea kettle with water and bring to a boil. Let eggs sit in kettle
about 12 minutes after the kettle shuts off.
Remove eggs and run cold water over egg shell for 1 minute.
Tap egg on hard surface to crack it, and then peel the shell. Add egg to large bowl.
Add onion, salt and pepper in mixing bowl.
Scoop out half an avocado and add to mixture.
Add mustard and mix well.
Serve on whole grain or sprouted grain bread, in wrap.
Egg salad also goes great over a salad!

Almond Butter & Fruit Pita
Equipment: None

Ingredients

    1/2 banana, sliced
    1/4 cup fresh strawberries, sliced
    2 pieces of your favorite whole grain or gluten-free pita bread (or Ezekiel wrap)
    2 Tbsp. almond butter mixed with 1 Tbsp. chia seeds

Directions

Split pita bread open.
Smear almond butter inside and pack with banana and strawberry slices.

Chickpea Walnut Bowl
Equipment: Can opener

Ingredients
    6 oz. chick peas (garbanzo beans), rinsed
    1 handful baby spinach
    1 handful kale
    1/2 cucumber, sliced (optional)
    1/4 chopped onion (optional)
    1/2 tomato, chopped – or 6 cherry tomatoes
    1/2 cup chopped walnuts
    6 sliced strawberries
    4 oz. goat cheese crumbles (optional)

Directions
Add kale and spinach to large bowl.

Combine remaining ingredients in bowl and drizzle with olive oil and balsamic vinegar.

This is a great recipe with which to experiment. Personally, I love adding raisins or grapes into most of my salads. I also sprinkle most everything with hemp and chia seeds. They're my go-to power pellets!

Chocolate Peanut Butter Sandwich
Equipment: None

Ingredients
    3 Tbsp. peanut butter
    2 Tbsp. hazelnut butter
    2 pieces of Ezekiel bread (toasted, if possible)

Directions
Spread peanut butter and hazelnut butter on whole grain bread.
This is a high-energy meal!

(For a lighter snack: Instead of bread, put these butters in the creases of celery!)

Grape & Lentil Salad
Equipment: Can opener

Ingredients
    1 cup black lentils, rinsed and drained
    1/2 cup grapes, halved
    2 cups power greens (spinach and kale, chopped)
    1/3 cup goat cheese (optional)
    1/2 tomato, sliced
    sprinkle of hemp seeds
    Dressing: light drizzle of extra virgin olive oil and balsamic vinegar

Directions
In a large bowl, add power greens, followed by grapes, lentils, cheese and tomato slices. Sprinkle with hemp seeds. Drizzle with olive oil and vinegar. This also is great in a wrap!

Honey & Nut Butter Sandwich
Equipment: None

Ingredients
    1 slice whole grain or gluten-free bread (toasted, if possible)
    1/2 tsp. honey or agave
    2 Tbsp. almond butter (or your favorite nut butter)

Directions
Spread honey and almond butter on bread and serve.

Mike's Avocado Salmon Salad
Equipment: Can opener

Ingredients
4 oz. wild-caught Alaskan Sockeye
1/2 stalk celery, chopped
1/4 cup red or sweet onion, chopped
2 tsp. spicy brown mustard or horseradish
2 Tbsp. dill pickle relish (unsweetened)
1/4 tsp. black pepper
7 pitted black olives, chopped (optional)
1/2 avocado
brown rice wrap or bread

Directions
Put salmon in a large mixing bowl and mash in celery, onion, mustard, relish, olives, pepper and avocado. Mix thoroughly, mashing avocado into the mixture. Transfer mixture to brown rice wrap or bread.

No-Cook Fighter Fajitas
Equipment: None

Ingredients
    4 oz. chicken breast*, packaged or grilled from cafeteria
    *(leave out for vegan option)
    1/2 cup black beans, rinsed (increase to 1 cup for vegan option)
    1/2 tsp. sea salt
    handful of baby spinach
    1/2 tsp. black pepper
    1 tomato, diced
    1 whole grain or gluten-free wrap
    1/4 avocado

Directions
Smear avocado onto wrap and then add remaining ingredients. Fold and eat!

Phenom Chicken & Date Wraps
Equipment: None

Ingredients
    4 oz. chicken breast, packaged or grilled from cafeteria
    1 whole grain or gluten-free wraps
    6 dates, pitted & sliced
    6 oz. small curd plain cottage cheese

Directions
Spread thin layer of cottage cheese on wraps and line with dates and chicken. That's it! Wrap and eat!

Strawberry Wrap
Equipment: None

Ingredients
2 handfuls baby spinach
10 fresh strawberries, sliced
1/2 avocado, cut into bite-sized chunks
1 cup crushed walnuts
1 whole grain or gluten-free wrap
light drizzle of extra virgin olive oil (optional)

Directions
Arrange spinach, avocado, walnuts and strawberries in a wrap. Drizzle with half a teaspoon of olive oil. Fold up and eat!

Tuna Stuffed Tomatoes
Equipment: None

Ingredients
2 large vine-ripened tomatoes
1 can tuna in water, drained
1/2 avocado or 2 Tbsp. Vegenaise
dash of black pepper

Directions
Wash and core tomatoes and set aside. In a small bowl, combine tuna, avocado (or Vegenaise) and pepper. Mix well. Stuff tuna mixture into tomatoes.

Warrior Salad
Equipment: None

Ingredients
    1/2 cup chopped walnuts
    1/2 cup plain Greek yogurt
    1/2 avocado
    1 tsp. honey
    dash of black pepper
    1 large apple, chopped into 1/2 inch pieces
    1/2 celery stalk, chopped
    1/3 cup raisins
    1/2 lemon, juiced
    2 handfuls baby spinach, chopped

Directions
Mix yogurt, avocado, honey and pepper in a bowl. Add the apple, celery and raisins and sprinkle with the lemon juice; toss with yogurt mixture. Wait to add walnuts and spinach until you're ready to eat the salad.

Apple with Nut Butter
Equipment: None

Ingredients
    1-2 Tbsp. of your favorite nut butter
    1 apple, whole or sliced (also try this with a banana!)

Directions
Dip apple slices (or smear on) the nut butter of your choice!
This is a great on-the-go-snack! **DolceDietShop.com** has excellent resources for finding inexpensive, high quality nut butters in single serve and bulk.

Black Bean Hummus
Equipment: Can opener

Ingredients
1 can black beans, rinsed and drained
1 garlic clove, chopped (substitute with garlic powder in a pinch!)
2 Tbsp. lemon juice
splash of water
vegetables for dunking

Directions
Blend (or smash with a fork really good!) the beans with the garlic, and lemon juice.
If mixture is too thick, splash some water in there and mix until desired consistency is reached.
Sprinkle with sea salt.
Serve with vegetables for dipping or roll onto a wrap for a great on-the-go snack.

Blueberry Madness
Equipment: None

Ingredients
    6 oz. plain Greek yogurt
    1/2 cup blueberries
    1 Tbsp. agave or honey
    1 tsp. chia seeds
    1 tsp. hemp seeds

Directions
Combine all ingredients in bowl and serve!

Coconut Fruit Cups
Equipment: None

Ingredients
1/2 banana
6 strawberries
1/2 cup chia seeds
handful of grapes
1/2 cup shredded unsweetened coconut

Directions
Combine ingredients in large bowl and mix well.
Put into small serving bowls.
Let sit for about 15 minutes, or until thickened.

Dates & Pecans
Equipment: None

Ingredients
4-6 dates, pitted
handful of pecans

Directions
Eat separately or combine in a bowl.

Almonds & Olives
Equipment: None

Ingredients
  3/4 cup almonds
  1/2 cup whole olives, pitted

Directions
Serve almonds and olives in two separate small bowls for the perfect complementary snack.

Stoned Grapes
Equipment: Freezer

Ingredients
   2 cups red grapes

Directions
Freeze for one hour (or more). They turn out like hard candies!
This is the perfect snack for when the munchies have you by the balls! Buy 2 lbs. of red grapes every week. Break them down in 6 oz. baggies and put them in your freezer. Makes an absolutely delicious and satisfying cold crunchy sugary treat. No more late night trips to Ben & Jerry's!

Power Pudding
Equipment: None

Ingredients
    3 Tbsp. chia seeds
    3 Tbsp. hemp seeds
    3 Tbsp. raisins
    1 cup water
    dash of cinnamon

Directions
Combine raisins, chia and hemp seeds in a large bowl with water.
Set aside for about 15 minutes or until thick.
Sprinkle with cinnamon.

This is great as a post-workout or anytime snack, full meal or dessert. I make a big bowl (four times bigger than this recipe calls for) and keep it in my refrigerator. That way, I'm able to scoop out as much as needed and store the rest.

Simple Guacamole Dip
Equipment: None

Ingredients
  2 large, ripe avocados, scooped out
  1/4 tomato, chopped
  2-3 Tbsp. lime juice, to taste
  1/3 cup onion, chopped
  1/2 tsp. chili powder, to taste
  1/2 tsp. sea salt
  chopped jalapeños (optional)
  vegetables for dipping

Directions
Combine all ingredients in mixing bowl and mash with fork to desired consistency.
Dip your favorite veggies!

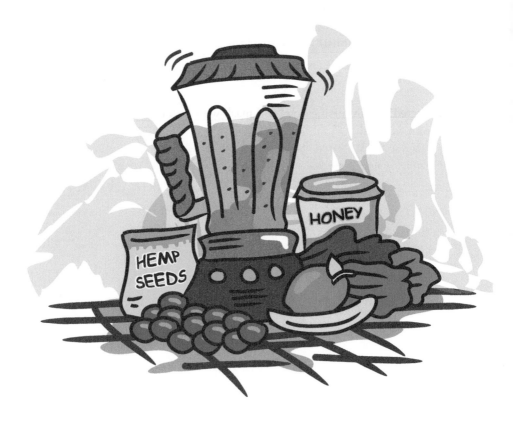

★ SMOOTHIES & DRINKS ★

These are some of the easiest, fastest, cheapest and tastiest on-the-go meals to make. Pop them into a travel mug and enjoy on the way to class! We've listed a few for you here, but always experiment. Remember to add in appetite sustaining, slow digesting ingredients like hemp seed and chia seed to keep your hunger in check and your energy high!

Green Tea GO! Drink
Equipment: Blender

Ingredients
8 oz. water
2 Tbsp. hemp seeds
2 Tbsp. chia seeds
1 green tea bag
1 tsp. honey or agave
1 cup frozen blueberries
1/2 banana
3/4 cup almond milk

Directions
Brew 8 oz. (regular coffee mug size) of green tea and stir in honey or agave and set aside.
Add all ingredients to the blender, green tea last.
Blend until creamy.

Oats & Berries Smoothie
Equipment: Blender

Ingredients
    1 cup blueberries
    1 cup strawberries
    2 Tbsp. hemp seeds
    2 Tbsp. chia seeds
    1/3 cup uncooked oat bran (or buckwheat)
    1/2 cup almond milk
    1/2 cup water

Directions
Combine in blender until creamy.

Peanut Butter Berry Drink
Equipment: Blender

Ingredients
1/2 banana
1/2 cup almond milk
2 Tbsp. hemp seeds
2 Tbsp. chia seeds
1/2 cup blueberries
1/2 cup strawberries
1 Tbsp. almond butter or peanut butter
1 tsp. honey or agave

Directions
Add all ingredients in the blender and process until thick.

WANT MORE RECIPES?
The Dolce Diet: Living Lean Cookbook features more than 130 Dolce Diet approved meals, and our free member site – **MyDolceDiet.com** – has a popular recipe group where you can exchange ideas with health-minded people from all over the world.

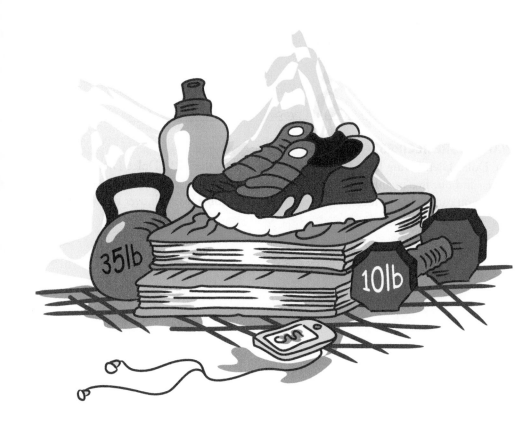

JAILHOUSE WORKOUTS

(Locked in Your Dorm Room)

You don't think a guy with a 21-inch neck and a 535-lb. bench press would spend an entire book talking about hemp seeds and doing your homework and not talk about adding slabs of thick muscle to your toned and tight physique, do you? Ladies, this goes for you, too! College is the time for all of you guys and girls to get out there and flaunt your bangin' bodies before the stress of the job you're working so hard to get makes it much more difficult. Lucky are you who can spend your days expanding your brain and spend your nights – well, bangin' away.

First, get yourself some weights. I don't care if they're your sister's pink Jane Fonda dumbbells. Put those bastards in your suitcase and get them in your dorm room. Wal-Mart sells weights for $1 per lb. That's right. You can get two 5 lb. dumbbells in your hands and start ripping out side lateral and bicep curls while waiting for your game to load on Xbox.

Now, here are a few flab-fighting, muscle-building workout routines to battle the beer gut and keep your mind sharp.

From the simple 3-minute workout I often use when traveling to the much more complex S.E.A.L. workout, all of these training routines can be implemented into your life, no matter how crazy your class schedule!

Note: Video examples of these exercises can be viewed at **CollegeDietGuide.com**.

1-MINUTE SPRINTS

Allocate 3 minutes per day: 1 minute in the morning, afternoon and night. Sounds very simple. Almost too simple to even attempt but do read on.

Morning: Bodyweight Squats for 60 seconds nonstop.
Afternoon: Push-ups for 60 seconds nonstop.
Night: V-ups for 60 seconds nonstop.

Write your reps down to keep track of your progress.

Week 1: Your first goal will be one rep every 2 seconds or 30 reps of each per day for 1 minute.

Week 2: One rep per second for 1 minute, or 60 reps of each per day for 1 minute.
Week 3: As many as you can do in 1 minute. Goal is 100 reps.
I like to keep a stop watch in front of me, whether it's the wall clock or my iPad on the floor, so I know where I stand.

CARDIO IN YOUR DORM

Jog in place. Nelson Mandela famously worked himself up to running a full marathon, while never leaving his jail cell. To pass the time and keep his mind and body sharp, Mandela would run in place with vigorous exertion for hours on end, completing the equivalent of many marathons. The lesson here: Where there is a will, there is a way. Start slow and build your base. In order for cardio to be effective, we must elevate our heart rate for 20 to 45 minutes.

Start at a very light 20-minute jog in place. Each day add 1 minute to your training time. At the end of 3 weeks, you'll be running over 40 minutes per session. This is the equivalent of 4 miles!

OUTDOOR CAMPUS WORKOUTS

JUMP ROPE

High Intensity Interval Training (HIIT) is a great way to get in shape. Keep a jump-rope (CollegeDietGuide.com) in your backpack and you can do it anywhere. Jumping rope is great for fat loss, metabolism stimulation and cardiovascular endurance, and it's inexpensive!

I like the On-Off Program – where we increase our ON time (training) and decrease our OFF time (rest).

Week 1: 30 seconds of jump rope and 30 seconds of rest for 10 minutes.
Week 2: 45 seconds of jump rope and 15 seconds of rest for 15 minutes.
Week 3: 5 minutes of jump rope and 1 minute of rest for 15 minutes or three, 5-minute rounds. (That's the equivalent of a full UFC fight!)

BIKE

If you have a bike, get on it and pedal! You determine the course.
Everything should be done in 3-week cycles. Set new goals for speed, distance, hills or terrain. Have fun and go!

WALK CAMPUS

Take it upon yourself to view your daily routine as a workout waiting to happen. I travel a heck of a lot. I'm on 2 to 10 airplanes per week and some days on 2 a day! I know I'll be doing a lot of walking through airports and unfamiliar terrain, so I wear active clothes made of dry-fit fabric and push the pace. Your walk to and from class is a mini cardio session! You don't need to break a sweat here, just push yourself in a manner more like hiking.

SPRINT STAIRS

Many schools have stairs, sports stadiums or bleachers. Heck, my wrestling room only had access to 16 stairs but that didn't stop me from using them for my purpose of getting fit. A minimum of 20-40 minutes per stair workout is perfect. Find your stairs and start stepping!

Some simple stair workouts:
    Jog the stairs for time.
    Sprint up, walk down.
    Single leg, single stair hop-ups.
    Single leg, double stair hop-ups.

BODY-PART SPECIFIC WORKOUTS

CHEST WORKOUT
I had great success building my chest by performing the following routine:
1 set of 20 push-ups when I woke up.
1 set of 30 push-ups before breakfast.
1 set of 50 push-ups 15 minutes after breakfast.
100 push-ups just before dinner.

That is 1,400 push-ups in 1 week! I bet that's 1,399 more push-ups than you did last week!

Types of Push-ups: Wide/Close/Medium

Standard push-up: I prefer elbows at 45 degrees to the body with elbows over wrists and on dumbbells to save the flexion in my wrists.

Try these alternate push-up styles:
- Feet wide
- Feet close
- One foot off the floor
- Feet elevated on chair
- Hands elevated on text books

ARMS
The following hi-rep exercises are where those pink dumbbells come in really handy. There are hundreds of combinations and exercises for arms.

I like to do what I call 99's – that's one regular curl, one hammer curl, and one reverse curl (palms up, thumbs up, knuckles up).

Here are more of my favorite arm exercises that require very little space and work great with hi-rep sets. I do exercises like these during commercial breaks of television shows or between rounds of fights, or while waiting for my team to get their shit together in the Xbox game lobby:

- Zottman curls
- Drag curls, which will help strengthen and build out the shoulder
- Overhead shoulder tricep presses
- Trap raises
- Laterals
- Close grip chest presses

SIMPLE LOWER BODY WORKOUT ROUTINE

Here is an example of a 3-week workout cycle. Use this as a foundation to create your own! Start with bodyweight squats, standard push-ups and V-ups. Use more challenging alternatives in future cycles (i.e. single leg squats, close-grip push-ups, etc.).

Cycle One

Week 1 – Everyday
3 sets x 10 reps
20 second break between all sets
Bodyweight Squats
Standard Push-ups
V-ups

Week 2 – Everyday
3 sets x 15 reps
15 second break between all sets
Bodyweight Squats
Standard Push-ups
V-ups

Week 3 – Everyday
5 sets x 20 reps
20 second break between all sets
Bodyweight Squats
Standard Push-ups
V-ups

Cycle Two

Week 1 – Everyday
5 sets x 10 reps
20 second break between all sets
Bodyweight Squats
Standard Push-ups
V-ups

Week 2 – Everyday
    5 sets x 15 reps
    15 second break between all sets
    Bodyweight Squats
    Standard Push-ups
    V-ups

Week 3 – Everyday
    5 sets x 20 reps
    20 second break between all sets
    Bodyweight Squats
    Standard Push-ups
    V-ups

GYM OR TRAINING FACILITY WORKOUTS

PUSH-PULL WORKOUTS

I prefer to think in terms of motions and not muscles. If I perform a deadlift, I am training my pull muscles; hamstrings, lower back, glutes, upper back and traps. Sometimes, it makes sense to train these muscle groups together. The same holds true for the push muscles of the chest, delts, triceps, quads and calves. This workout is appropriate for novices, women, health-minded individuals and professional athletes. These are the very same workouts my world-class athletes perform. Give them a try and see how you fare.

PUSH WORKOUT

Overhead Squat
2 sets x 20 reps warm up
5 sets x 12 reps
-60 seconds rest between sets.
-60 seconds rest between exercises.

Incline Dumbbell Press
2 sets x 20 reps warm up
3 sets x 12 reps
-20 seconds rest between sets.
-45 seconds rest between exercises.

Dumbbell Front Laterals
3 sets x 15 reps
-20 seconds rest between sets.
-45 seconds rest between exercises.

Close-Grip Bosu Ball Push-up
5 sets x 10 reps
-20 seconds rest between sets.
-45 seconds rest between exercises.

X-Pattern Toe Touch
2 sets x 50 reps (each side)
-30 seconds rest between each set.

PULL WORKOUT

Two-Arm Bent-Over Dumbbell Row
2 sets x 20 reps warm up
5 sets x 8 reps
-60 seconds rest between sets.
-60 seconds rest before next exercise.

High-Hip Barbell Deadlift
1 set x 20 reps - warm up
1 set x 10 reps - warm up
1 set x 5 reps - bridge set
5 sets x 5 reps - work sets

*This workout might look like this:
135 x 20 / 185 x 10 / 225 x 5 / 275 x 5 x 5

-60 seconds rest between sets.
-Practice deep breathing between each set.
-Rest 60 seconds before next exercise.

Single Leg Dumbbell Deadlift
3 sets x 10 reps
-60 seconds rest between sets.
-60 seconds rest before next exercise.

Barbell Upright Row
3 sets x 15 reps
-60 seconds rest between sets.

Alternate Straight-Leg Crunch
5 sets x 20 reps (each side)
-30 seconds rest between each set.

TANK TOP WORKOUT
This workout is great for ladies looking to tighten and tone or elite athletes looking to maximize upper body endurance. Sets and reps for beginners should be reduced until a mastery of form is achieved.

Bosu Ball Push-up
5 sets x 15 reps
-30 seconds rest between each set.
-60 seconds rest between each exercise.

Barbell Bench Press
1 set x 100 reps with empty bar
-30 seconds rest between each set.
-60 seconds rest between each exercise.

Barbell Upright Row
3 sets x 20 reps
-30 seconds rest between each set.
-60 seconds rest between each exercise.

Dumbbell Side Laterals
3 sets x 20 reps
-30 seconds rest between each set.
-60 seconds rest between each exercise.

Incline Bench Triceps Extension
2 sets x 30 reps
-30 seconds rest between each set.
-60 seconds rest between each exercise.

Bosu Ball Push-up
2 sets to failure
-60 seconds rest between sets.

THE FIGHTER'S TREADMILL WORKOUT
Warm up
5 minute walk at 3 mph

Round 1
1 minute at 8 mph
1 minute at 6 mph
1 minute at 8 mph
1 minute at 6 mph
1 minute at 8 mph
1 minute walk at 3 mph

Round 2
1 minute at 9 mph
1 minute at 6 mph

1 minute at 9 mph
1 minute at 6 mph
1 minute at 9 mph
1 minute walk at 3 mph

Round 3
1 minute at 10 mph
1 minute at 6 mph
1 minute at 10 mph
1 minute at 6 mph
1 minute at 10 mph

Cool-down
5 minute walk at 3 mph

Goal: All three rounds at 10 mph during sprint interval.

S.E.A.L. WORKOUT

For those who want a greater challenge, this workout is based upon the necessary physical requirements to even think about thinking about being a Navy S.E.A.L.

500 Yard Swim – perform under 12 minutes, 30 seconds. Goal: 8-9 minutes.
Push-ups – perform a minimum of 42 in 2 minutes. Goal: 100.
Sit-ups – perform a minimum of 52 in 2 minutes. Goal: 100.
Pull-ups – perform a minimum of 8 with no limit. Goal: 20.
1.5 Mile timed run – perform under 11 minutes, 30 seconds. Goal: 9-10 minutes.

This is just a start! There are a million workouts that can be done in your room, outside around campus or in your school's gym. The key is to find one that keeps you motivated!

Note: Check out **CollegeDietGuide.com** for examples of these exercises.

RIDGE

Age: 23 · **Starting Weight:** 170 · **Current Weight:** 155

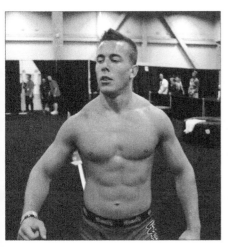 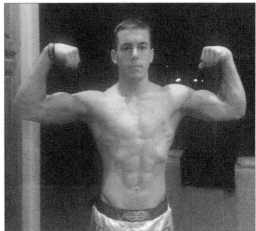

I wrestled at 133 lbs. in 2011 and 2012 for the University of Nebraska. Within 5 months of the 2012 season I weighed 170 lbs. with only 6.5 percent body fat, and had outgrown multiple weight classes. Going into my fifth and final year, I wanted to compete at 149 lbs. or 157 lbs. but the team was strongest with me at 141 lbs. This is where Mike Dolce came in.

I ordered Living Lean and 3 Weeks to Shredded. Over the course of 1 month, I was able to shrink my body from 165 to 141 lbs. while feeling great!

During the season, I was able to maintain a healthy range for my weight class, which resulted in a fairly easy weight cut every week. I am continuing to Live Lean by applying Mike's nutritional principles, and will continue to do so the rest of my life. I wish I had followed these principles earlier in my career because it would have made a huge difference. I underperformed at times because of unhealthy weight cutting habits. Mike's knowledge could help change the wrestling world!"

Note: Ridge graduated with a B.S. in Business Administration. He now owns Unrivaled Sports Performance in Lincoln, Nebraska — a DOLCE APPROVED training facility.

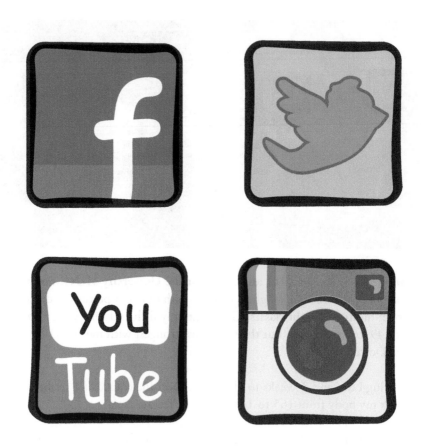

MORE RESOURCES

COLLEGEDIETGUIDE.COM
CollegeDietGuide.com is your one-stop resource for everything mentioned in this book, including free grocery and equipment list downloads, meal ideas and more! Be sure to take a peek in between classes!

THEDOLCEDIET.COM
Check out **TheDolceDiet.com** for up-to-date news items and blogs from Mike detailing recipes, workout tips, videos and behind-the-scenes content with the world's most elite athletes.

MYDOLCEDIET.COM
Visit **MYDolceDiet.com** for your free profile page! Talk directly with Mike during his frequent LIVE CHATS, and connect with others just like yourself to share tips, recipes and join support groups.

TWITTER @TheDolceDiet
Follow Mike on **Twitter.com/TheDolceDiet** and be sure to join in on his live Q&A sessions each Sunday!

FACEBOOK
Check out The Dolce Diet fan page at **Facebook.com/TheDolceDiet**

YOUTUBE
Be sure to visit The Dolce Diet YouTube channel at **YouTube.com/dolcediet** for videos detailing exercises, recipes and so much more!

INSTAGRAM
See what fun and informative subjects Mike's taking pictures of today on Instagram at **instagram.com/thedolcediet**